Facial Exercis Easy For a Youthful Look

Step By Step Guide to Facial Exercises to Tone and Firm Up Your Face Muscles for A Youthful Look

Introduction

Do you have wrinkles and want to firm up your skin?

Or

Have you tried to tighten and firm up your skin for a young youthful look, but nothing seems to work?

If the above statements describe you, then you've come to the right place.

<u>You Are About To Discover A Step By Step Guide To Facial Exercises To Tone And Firm Up Your Face Muscles For a Youthful Look</u>

According to experts, doing a few facial exercises a day can do wonders for your skin, and this book will take you through simple facial exercises you can do to improve your skin and firm it up for a younger look.

Here is a preview of what you will find in the book:

In it, you will find:

- What are facial exercises and face yoga

- The scientific reasoning behind facial exercises and face yoga

- Benefits of doing facial exercises

- How you can effortlessly prepare for face yoga

- Tons of Facial exercises targeting your forehead, eyebrows, eyelids, cheeks and mouth, your lips, the chin, neck, and even more!

- Cool-down: What to do after practicing facial exercises

And much, much more!

The time for you to start facial workouts and face yoga is NOW.

Let us get started!

PS: I'd like your feedback. If you are happy with this book, please leave a review on Amazon.

Please leave a review for this book on Amazon by visiting the page below:

https://amzn.to/2VMR5qr

Table of Contents

Facial Exercises in a Nutshell

The concept behind facial exercises is that they tone, lift, and boost the volume of facial muscles. In fact, these exercises work similarly to regular exercises that often target the quads or biceps.

Further, according to <u>scientific studies</u>[1], facial exercises can help make your skin look younger, all while giving you firmer and fuller lower and upper cheeks. The findings were from a 5-month study that involved 16 women aged between 40 and 60 years.

In the study, participants undertook 90-minute training sessions with the direct supervision of a trained yoga instructor. After the first eight weeks of training, participants undertook daily yoga exercises and progressed to an alternate-day facial exercise routine at 12 weeks.

During the study, researchers took photos of the women at three intervals: first, at the beginning of the study, at week 8,

---

[1]

<u>https://jamanetwork.com/journals/jamadermatology/fullarticle/266680</u><u>1</u>

and after 20 weeks of exercise. At the program's start, dermatologists reviewed participants' photos and rated them ass 50.8 years through standardized facial aging scales.

By week 12, a similar review indicated that participants looked exactly 49.1 years old, almost three years younger! In a related study[2] where participants completed 30 minutes of daily facial exercises for 20 weeks, researchers experienced the same results.

All these studies show one thing with absolute certainty, facial exercises work and can do wonders for your skin once you start practicing them consistently.

The following chapter will focus on some benefits of doing facial exercises:

---

[2]

https://jamanetwork.com/journals/jamadermatology/fullarticle/2666801

Benefits of Facial Exercises

Below are some benefits you stand to gain from by doing facial exercises:

Tighter, fuller, plumper skin

Doing regular facial exercises helps contour the face, reduce lines and shape it. The exercises also help boost blood flow, release tension, and can further increase your facial glow.

Reduces signs of aging

Just like body exercises strengthen different body muscles, facial exercises strengthen different facial muscles. Facial exercises help strengthen the muscles below the skin and facilitate the growth of fuller lower and upper cheeks, making you look quite younger.

Boosts facial muscles strength

We lose a significant amount of collagen as we age, resulting in wrinkles, sagging, and skin drooping. Doing facial workouts allows you to build face muscles that help plump up spots that would otherwise show reduced collagen levels signs.

Particularly, facial exercises help plump up the cheek area. Once you thoroughly workout the facial muscles, facial movement increases heat and micro-circulation in the muscles, making them stronger and firmer.

However, as a beginner, you're likely to feel a bit tired after a few minutes of exercising, but this should go away with time.

Note:

Before you begin, ensure you apply a little moisturizer to your face. It's also best to rub the moisturizer into your fingertips too. This helps stop any possible pulling or tearing of the skin.

Let us now look at some exercises you can do, based on where they target:

Facial Exercises For The Forehead

These facial exercises workout the forehead area:

Forehead Fine-Tuning

This exercise helps smooth face lines and wrinkles from your forehead, and the best thing is that you can practice it almost everywhere without making weird faces!

- Try acting surprised for a few seconds.

- Keep your forehead a bit frozen as much as you can while widening your eyes to the fullest

- Then repeat the pose about 8 to 10 times a day for a few weeks until you get your desired outcome.

Forehead Workout

- First, put your finger on both your eyelids to set them in place, and then raise your brows.

- Repeat this exercise for 10 rounds until you get used to the workout; you should manage to do it without using your fingers. Now gaze straight ahead and begin pulling your forehead tight as if you want to bring it back over the top of your head.

- Hold this pose for about 10 seconds and then repeat.

- At this point, get to a more advanced forehead workout. Pull your forehead back as done in the previous exercise, and try lifting your brow from each eye individually.

- Repeat the exercise approximately 10 times per eyebrow.

"Rubber" Exercise for forehead

This workout helps reduce those horizontal wrinkles appearing on your forehead.

- To begin with, wrap your hands at the back of your head.

- Now place your hands on the hairline border of your forehead.

- Then pull yourself a little bit backward using your hands.

- At this point, pulse your lips to form the letter "O" shape and then look down. Hold this pose for approximately 10 seconds or so.

- Repeat the rubber exercise for about 20 rounds. Be aware that the exercise can create tension in your forehead.

Forehead Push With Your Hands

Here, you will use your hands to trigger resistance as you flex the brows. By doing so, you'll get smooth lines on the forehead.

- Position each of your palms on the sides of the forehead, while the bottom of individual palms lies on your brows.

- Ensure your palms can strongly hold your skin in place.

- Now raise your eyebrow muscles and then quickly lower them in a frowning pose.

- Just raise and lower the eyebrows for ten rounds, and then raise and hold the pose for approximately 30 seconds.

- Then lower the eyebrows and likewise hold the pose for another 30 seconds.

- At this point, repeat the raising and lowering exercise for another ten rounds.

Forehead and Eyes Exercise

This exercise helps smooth those visible lines on your forehead.

- To practice this exercise, begin by pulling your forehead using your index finger.

- Now apply pressure on the forehead with just the fingers so you can strengthen the face as your eyebrows shift in position.

- Position your index fingers just over each eye and then pull down on them as you attempt to raise your brows.

- Repeat the exercise for about ten rounds or until you feel tension on your forehead.

The Forehead Palm Stroke

This exercise helps relieve tension from your forehead's frontalis muscle. Once you relax this muscle, there's a reduced likelihood of creating an expression on your forehead, which also boosts circulation and tightens your skin.

- To practice this exercise, your forehead needs to relax fully, and your eyebrows shouldn't move up or down. You can choose to either open or close your eyes.

- Now put one palm on the middle of your forehead and then strike the palm of your hand across.

- Now lift the palm off and use the other palm of your hand to slide the initial hand in the opposite direction.

- Repeat this pose for approximately 1 minute as you alternate hands in different strokes, taking care not to drag your skin forcefully.

- Take a few minutes to experience how it feels to have a relaxed forehead. You can then repeat the palm stroke exercise anytime you feel off balance.

The Forehead Walk

This exercise can help balance your mind while brightening your forehead area. Doing this soothes acupressure points which helps relax tense muscles and reduce the expression of lines on your forehead.

- Evenly space your index, ring, and middle fingers of both hands on your brows.

- Then press the eyebrows while taking a deep breath through your nose.

- Now move the forehead to the hairline approximately 1 centimeter at each movement, as you take a deep breath with each press for about 10 seconds or so.

- Repeat the exercise for another round of 30 seconds.

- You might experience a little bit of redness on your forehead due to increased blood flow to the skin. Take care not to press the top layer of skin too hard.

21

Forehead pose

This pose helps remove the frown lines or the horizontal wrinkles that appear on your face.

- First, put the tips of your fingers just over the eyebrows.

- Then, begin lifting your eyebrows as much as you can as you simultaneously press the skin with your fingertips downwards to help block movement.

- Hold this yoga pose for about 6 to 10 seconds and then do another 5 to 10 repetitions.

Smooth The Brow For Forehead:

This yoga pose is suitable for horizontal forehead lines and works similarly to Botox.

- Put both hands facing inwards on your forehead and then spread the fingers out between the hairline and your eyebrows.

- Slowly sweep all your fingers outwards **across** your forehead, and apply a little pressure to tighten the skin.

- Relax and repeat this exercise for ten rounds.

Exercises for The Eyes and Eyebrows

The following facial exercises will work out your eyes and eyebrows:

Eye-firming Cheek Plumper

- Put both hands horizontally just under your lower lash line and just above your cheekbones.

- Put your index fingers under your lashes, and then position the little fingers under your cheekbones.

- Now press your hands on the surface of your skin to hold the muscles in place.

- Then squint your eyes as you squeeze your cheeks up to the direction of your eyes as if you want to make a squishy sour face.

- Hold this position for a count of 5 and do 3 to 5 repetitions.

Wink n' Hold

This exercise helps reduce lines and wrinkles from your under the eye region.

- Wink a little bit, and then hold the partial wink for a few seconds.

- Ensure you contract all the muscles around the winked eye, then release the pose slowly.

- Repeat the exercise approximately 20 to 25 times per set in a day.

- Do not overdo the exercise.

Brow Raiser

This exercise can help perk up your eyebrows and keep them in their position, especially due to constant wincing and aging, which can make the eyebrows droop.

Here's how you can get those taut eyebrows within a few weeks:

- First, stick both your index and middle finger together.

- Then, put the fingers a few millimeters from your eyebrows and gently start pushing the skin down.

- Force your eyebrows to go up and down as you gradually add tension with your fingers and push down.

- Repeat the exercise for six sets of 10 brows raises and drops on each set.

Eye Toning

If you have droopy eyelids, here are great exercises that also work well for eye bags, crow's feet, and puffiness.

- Put your middle and index fingers in a V shape on your eyes.

- Then press and hold down the fingers together around the inner corner of your eyebrows.

- Gaze up, raise your lower eyelids upward to create a strong squint and then relax.

- Repeat the exercise about six additional times.

- To end your set, firmly squeeze your eyes shut for approximately 10 seconds.

Droopy Eyes and Crow's Feet Exercise

- Position your middle fingers in between your eyebrows.

- Set your index fingers beside the outer corner of your eyes.

- Slowly move your index finger upwards and then outwards. Now, look up.

- Hold this position for around 4 seconds and then release.

- Repeat the exercise for a set of 5 rounds continuously.

Eyes Workout

This exercise helps alleviate eye bags and boosts blood flow to reduce dark circles.

- First, close your eyes. You can also hold them closed if that's comfortable for you.

- Now raise your brows as far as possible to contract and strengthen the eye muscles.

- At this point, face your mirror and then pull the muscles under the eye as far as possible. Try doing it without squinting.

Try keeping your eye as wide as possible while avoiding squinting, which can cause wrinkles.

Frown Line Smoother

This exercise boosts the relaxation of the procerus muscle located between your eyebrows. Its relaxation reduces the chances of eyebrows furrowing, which can help eliminate lines on the forehead. The exercise also helps boost blood, oxygen, and nutrients flow on the forehead.

- First, form your index fingers into small hooks.

- Now stroke along the muscle between your brows using your knuckles.

- Begin from the little dip on top of your nose and continue stroking up to the hairline.

- Continue with the stroking motion in an upward motion for about 1 minute or so.

- Take care not to press the muscle so hard or create extra pressure on your skin. You should feel a bit comfortable with the exercise.

The Flirty Eyes For Brows

This face exercise is suitable for drooping eyebrows and deep eye hollows; it can work as an eyebrow lift exercise.

- Position your index fingers below each of your eyes, pointing to the direction of your nose.

- Then, put your teeth under the lips and form an "O" shape with your mouth.

- Now flutter your upper eyelids as you gaze up for approximately 30 seconds.

Eyebrows Focus

This workout helps smooth your eyebrows.

- To exercise, first open your eyes as wide as possible while ensuring you don't form wrinkles on your eyebrows.

- Maintain this pose and try focusing on an imaginary point in the distance for around 15 seconds, and then relax.

- Repeat the exercise for another four rounds.

Eyebrow Stretch

This exercise helps firm the muscles around your eyebrows and eyes to reduce the puffiness, diminish crow's feet, and firm drooping eyelids.

- First, press your middle fingers together around the crown of your nose and at your brows' inner corner.

- Using your index fingers, firmly apply pressure to the corners of your brows.

- At this point, gaze towards the ceiling and lift your lower eyelids into a squint.

- Hold this pose for a couple of seconds, then relax.

- Repeat the workout for 5 rounds and then squeeze your eyes shut for approximately 15 seconds.

Exercises for The Lips and Nose

Here are effective facial exercises for the lips and nose:

Fish Lips

- Start by sucking your lips like a fish, with your lips pursed.

- With your lips still pursed, try smiling as hard as you can manage. Try your best to relax the other parts of your face, particularly the eyes.

- Hold this position for 10 seconds, and then relax.

- Try doing four repetitions a day.

Kiss Face

- Begin by pouting your lips as if you want to kiss someone.

- Try smiling with your lips pursed and relax your eyes.

- Hold the position for 10 seconds and then relax.

- Relax and repeat the kiss face exercise a total of four times a day.

The Whistler

- First, make an "O" shape with your lips as if you want to whistle.

- Try smiling very hard, with your lips forward in the initial pose "O."

- Relax and repeat the pose around three times or so.

- At this point, repeat the first two steps.

- Then, pump your cheek muscles up and down about 12 times with your lips in the previous "O" shape.

- Relax and repeat the last two steps about four times a day.

Lips Workout

This exercise helps strengthen sagging lip muscles, especially when done regularly.

- First, open your mouth wide, and then make the letter O.

- Hold this pose for approximately 3 seconds and then repeat.

- Practice the letter O exercise for ten rounds or longer. The idea is to feel comfortable when doing it, so workout until you can do it quickly and easily.

- Then put your thumbs below your top lip and now pull out slowly as you pull back with your jaw muscles simultaneously.

- The objective here is to pull your chin down as if you want to stretch your chin line.

- Repeat the exercise about ten times.

- Now open your mouth very wide and pull the muscles of the mouth sideways on your top lip.

Lines Around Your Nose

- Slightly open your mouth and then lift your top lip to the preferred side of the nose.

- You can try the exercise on both sides of the nose and then to one side at each exercise.

Normally it's easier doing it on one side, but it might be quite difficult to do one on the other side.

"Grandma" Workout For Lips

This exercise helps remove the nasolabial folds on your lips.

- Begin by opening your mouth wide.

- Then hide your lips under your jaws or teeth.

- Now tighten the pressure and then draw your lips inside the mouth.

- Hold this pose for 10 seconds, and then repeat for up to 15 rounds.

Squeeze Your Lips

This workout helps recondition the lip muscles. The rule of the thumb is to squeeze your face around your nose and mouth progressively.

- To begin, place your palms on your face such that the bottom edges are on top of your jawline and the outer edges are on your laugh line.

- Ensure you hold your face with your whole palm to ensure you exert enough pressure on the skin.

- Now push your lips together using your lip muscles and hold this pose for approximately 20 seconds.

- Then, push your palms up to the direction of your nose and now hold the pose for about 10 seconds.

- Repeat this squeezing exercise another three times.

Midface Pose

This pose is useful for the nasolabial fold lines on the sides of your nose that run to the corners of the mouth.

- First, open your mouth and then purse the lips to some extent.

- Then, place the index fingers of each hand against the corners of each side of the mouth.

- Now start protruding your lips as you pull the corners of your mouth outward, using your index fingers.

- Hold this pose for approximately 6 seconds, and do another 6 to 8 repetitions.

Fuller Lips Workout

This exercise helps make your lips appear fuller.

- Start with a sultry pout by moving your lips forward **far** enough **such that** the upper lip **can** touch the nose.

- Then turn both your lips inward and press them together, as if holding an object with the lips.

- Hold this pose for about 8 seconds, and repeat at least five more rounds.

Upper Lip Exercise

This facial workout helps remove the vertical lines that appear over your upper lips, also called lipstick lines.

- **Bring the** thumbs **from each hand** together while tucked up, and **then** place **them** together below your upper lip.

- Then, push the upper lip forward as you try to push your lip against your thumbs.

- Hold this pose for about 8 seconds, and then do around 5 to 10 reps.

Lip Pull

This exercise helps tone your facial muscle and gives you a toned jawline and high cheeks.

- Whether standing or sited, set your head facing straight and forward.

- Then lift your lower lip as you push your lower jaw out. Ensure that you can feel a stretch in your chin muscles.

- Hold this pose for a few seconds, relax for a minute and then repeat the exercise.

Exercises For the Cheeks

The following exercises will give you youthful-looking cheeks:

Cheekbone Lift

To get sharper cheekbones, follow these steps:

- Put together your middle and index fingers and position them over each cheekbone.

- Then gently lift the skin until you feel it slightly get tight.

- At this point, open your mouth into an oval shape "O" until you feel some resistance in your cheek muscles.

- Hold this pose for approximately 5 seconds or so.

- For defined cheekbones, repeat this exercise about 10 to 15 times

Cheek Plumping

This simple technique helps plump up your skin by raising the skin folds around the nose.

- Begin by smiling as hard as you can!

- Then, press down on the skin folds between your lips and nose using your fingertips.

- Gently raise your cheek muscles as you press down to trigger some resistance.

- Ensure your fingertips remain firm so that you don't over-stress your hand.

- Repeat the exercise for 2 to 3 minutes, with a few well-spaced rests.

Cheek Squeeze

This exercise helps eliminate flabby cheeks, giving you that slim, good-looking face.

- First, tilt your head all the way to your back.

- Then gently push your chin forward while taking care not to strain your neck.

- At this point, suck your cheeks in to create a fish face while being careful not to bite down on your tongue or lips.

- Repeat the exercise about 10 to 15 sets made up of 5 seconds of fish face per round.

The Cheek Lift

This smiling exercise helps you work out your lips and boosts your mood.

- First, close your lips slowly while pulling your cheeks in the direction of your eyes.

- Ensure you've raised the corner of your lips to the fullest and then smile widely.

- Now hold the pose for about 10 seconds.

Saxophone Cheeks

- Begin by closing your lips strongly.

- Then suck air through your mouth and now puff up your cheeks.

- Try holding the air in your right cheek for around 5 seconds, and then breathe out.

- Stitch the positions and now hold air in your left cheek, and then exhale.

- Repeat the exercise 10 times and then return to your initial pose.

Cheeks Workout

- For this exercise, try smiling as hard as you can go while you place your fingers on your cheekbones.

- Push down as hard as possible while maintaining your grin.

- Now face the mirror. Try grinning from only one side of your face as much as you can manage.

- Pull up the cheek muscle as much as possible and hold this pose for around 10 seconds or so.

- Repeat the exercise ten times, then change to the other cheek and start again.

Puffy Cheeks Exercise

This exercise helps reduce fat from both the middle and upper portions of your cheeks. In so doing, the facial exercise helps workout your upper cheek muscles while making your face well sculpted, young, and lean. To begin with:

- Close your mouth and then gently blow enough air to puff up your cheeks.

- Hold this position for 10 seconds.

- Then try moving the air from your left to your right cheek, and then hold the air for another 10 seconds or so.

- To complete the workout, blow air to your left cheek and hold the position for 10 seconds, then breathe out and relax for a few seconds.

- Repeat the exercise ten times.

Tightly Close The Eyes

This simple yet effective technique helps tone your cheeks to achieve that young look.

- To begin with, firmly close your eyes until you can feel some contraction in your facial muscles.

- Hold the pose for about 10 seconds, then relax your face. For consistent results, try doing the exercise a total of five times a day.

Stretch Your Face Muscles

This facial workout technique helps stretch your face muscles while working with your hands.

- To get started, lower your chin to the extent that it touches your chest.

- Then begin pulling the skin such that it comfortably moves underneath your cheekbones.

- Once you're in a fully relaxed position, start to pronounce the "Ah" sound.

- Maintain this pose for a few seconds and then relax.

- You should repeat the workout three times a day.

Blow Balloons

This exercise is a good way to tone as well as slim down your cheeks. Some reports from people who've used this exercise indicate that within five days, you'll begin to notice considerable changes in your chubby cheeks.

- First, get a balloon then proceed to inflate it. As you blow air in, take time to appreciate the pressure in your cheeks and how they expand.

- Then release the air from your balloon and repeat the blowing air exercise another ten times or so.

Rotating Tongue Exercise

This workout helps reduce the size of chubby cheeks since it reduces the amount of cheek fat.

- First, close your mouth, then rotate your tongue into gentle circular movements.

- As you rotate the tongue, ensure it touches the outer surface of your lower and upper teeth.

- Do the exercise approximately 15 times in both clockwise and anticlockwise directions.

Hot Towel Treatment

Regular facial steam treatment can effectively reduce your cheek fat as it triggers the face to sweat and release fats from the cheeks.

- First, boil some water, then transfer it into a bowl.

- Allow the water to cool down a little bit, then dip a towel.

- Slowly position the steaming towel onto the wrinkled and fatty areas of the face.

- Repeat the exercise five more times.

This exercise is best done 1 hour before bedtime. A facial steam workout helps open pores in your face and tone the skin.

Facial Exercises for The Jaw, Neck, and Shoulders

The following facial exercises will do wonders for your jaw, neck, and shoulders:

Jawline Workout

Often, the jawline is where you begin to notice saggy skin. To work out your jawline, you'll need to pull the jaw muscles forward and backward until you feel some stretching or elastic feeling.

Follow these steps:

- First, pull your jawline and lower cheeks away from the mouth.

- Maintain the mouth quite open, and now pull the lower half of your face into a grin or grimace.

- Try ignoring your cheekbones and only engage your jawline. Repeat this workout about ten times or so.

- At this point, try the exercise one side of the jaw at a time. Be aware that this might need more practice time but can produce better results.

- The rule of the thumb is to learn how to tighten your face muscles to an extent where you can practice anytime, whether at work or seated on the couch. Keep working until you can do the exercise much more quickly and easily.

Jaw-line Defined

- Put your hands together in a flat **fist**, position your chin over the hands, then press to create a resistance platform under the chin.

- Put your tongue on the roof of your mouth as you tuck your chin to your chest. Repeat this exercise for about five reps.

- Alternate this exercise with an open mouth, and drop your jaw and chin to your Do-It-Yourself platform.

- Repeat this exercise for about five reps, and hold the count for another five repetitions.

- Repeat the jawline for three sets as you alternate each movement.

The X and O Exercise

If you want to strengthen your jaw and neck muscles, this exercise triggers a lot of movement that helps burn fat in these regions.

- First, keep your head quite stiff and then relax your face.

- Try uttering Letters O and X such that your jaws, lips, and cheeks show a good movement.

- Try repeating this exercise approximately ten times and then relax.

Neck Workout

- To get that smooth neck, first, close your mouth and then gaze at the ceiling.

- Ensure you stretch your back as far as possible, and then put the lower lip over your top lip.

- Practice this work out several times until you find it easy to stretch further while at the same time placing your lower lip over the top lip and smiling to the maximum.

Neck Stretches

It's important to do neck stretches to relax. Let's begin with the simplest way to stretch neck muscles:

- To stretch the muscles located on the right side, turn the left ear over the left shoulder.

- Then hold for around 20 seconds or so. Repeat on the left side and turn the right ear this time around.

- Relax for some time, then roll the shoulder to the back. Then roll the front. Now lift your shoulders to the ears and let them drop completely as you tense the muscles.

- Repeat the neck exercise three more times.

Neck Mobilization Workout

This neck stretching workout is also called the "8 Corners":

- First, lift your head slightly off your pillow, then let the head follow the eyes while looking towards each corner of the house. Do not move your shoulders.

- Start with the corners of the ceiling first, and then follow the eyes to the flour to finish one round.

- Repeat ten times clockwise, eight corners represent one repetition (1 rep).

- Switch to the opposite direction and repeat for another ten repetitions. Ensure that the torso or shoulders do not move.

Jawline Pose

This workout helps exercise a double chin and a sagging jawline.

- First, position your elbow on a table with your fist placed under the chin.

- Press the chin upward with your fist as you try to open your jaw.

- Hold this pose for approximately 6 to 8 seconds and do another 5 to 10 repetitions.

Jaw Release

This exercise helps stretch the facial muscles around your lips, cheeks, and jaws.

- Choose to either sit or stand in a straight posture.

- Then move your jaw as if you are chewing, as you keep your lips closed.

- Breathe in deeply, then exhale while slowly humming.

- Next, open your mouth as wide as possible while pressing your tongue within your bottom teeth.

- Hold this pose for approximately 5 seconds, now inhale and exhale again.

- Repeat the workout about ten times.

Neck and Shoulders Stretches

To do a combined neck and shoulder stretch, do the following:

- Stand shoulder-width apart, and then raise your right arm to the shoulder height.

- Move the arm across the front of your body. Pull the right arm very close to the chest with your left arm.

- Hold for a moment, then switch arms and repeat.

- Do 3 to 5 sets of 30 seconds each to complete the shoulder stretch.

Another variation of the shoulder exercise is the "Upward Stretch."

- First, raise your arms towards the sky to help get your blood flowing to various organs.

- Then race fingers together and raise hands above your hand, with the palms facing upward.

- Gently elongate the spine and hold for a moment to feel the stretch in your arms and rib cage.

- Hold for a count of 10 and then relax and start again.

Shoulder Rolls

- To begin shoulder rolling, come up to a crawl position, preferably on your bed, shoulder placed over your hands.

- Maintain the elbows straight, then do clockwise circles using the shoulder blades.

- Repeat the exercise about 10-15 times, then switch directions

Exercises for the Chin

Here are the most effective chin workouts:

Double Chin Workout

A double chin forms because of the platysma muscle that links your jawline to the shoulders. Once the muscle gets loose, you get sagging skin around your neck.

Here is a simple exercise that helps straighten the platysma muscle to get a toned neck, jaw area, and chin!

- Whether seated or standing, gaze upwards and then tilt your head all the way to the back.

- Hold your head still, and then touch your tongue to the roof of your mouth. You might feel a little prickly pain in the neck as your muscles contract.

- Gently let go and now bring your chin down to its initial position. Repeat the exercise in a set of 5 rounds, each of the sets being approximately 25 to 30 seconds of tongue holding.

Pout and Tilt

This exercise is suitable for you if you have double chins.

- Begin seated in a straight posture.

- Then bend your head a bit backward.

- At this point, make a stiff pout and then hold this pose for approximately 10 seconds.

- Repeat the exercise for a set of 2 more rounds.

Double Chin Workout

- Twork out the double chin, first close your mouth, and then gaze at the sky or the ceiling.

- Then, make your mouth into an O shape and practice this a few times.

- Now change your mouth from letter O to a different letter E, and then back to O!

- Keep alternating the letters until you feel comfortable. Aim for about ten rounds of the workout.

"Hooligan" for Double Chin

This workout reduces the double chin while boosting the neck muscle tone.

- Remove your tongue from the mouth and point it upwards.

- Then turn your head slightly up, and slowly turn the head to the right.

- Now lift your chin and hold this pose for around 10 seconds.

- Return to the basic pose and repeat the steps in the opposite direction.

- Repeat the workout for about five rounds in each direction.

Mandibular Exercise For Double Chin

This workout helps strengthen your lower jaw, also called the mandible. This mandibular muscle is useful at preventing a double chin and physical signs of aging appearing on the lower part of your mouth.

- To practice, maintain your teeth and lips slightly closed.

- Then try separating your teeth as far as possible, taking care not to open your lips.

- Now bring your lower jaw forward gently as far as you can.

- Continue stretching your lower lip up, and hold this pose for approximately 5 seconds.

- Gently return your mandibles, lips, and teeth to the initial pose.

Chin Lifts

This exercise is great for getting rid of a double chin. It helps work out and stretch most facial muscles – this includes the muscles on the neck, throat and jaw. But make sure you do not use any other facial muscle other than the lips while doing this exercise. You can perform this exercise either in the sitting or standing position.

- Begin by tilting your head towards the ceiling, keeping your eyes fixed towards it.

- Now, make your lips tight, as if trying to kiss the ceiling, hold it to a count of 10 seconds and relax.

- Repeat this exercise a total of 10 times.

Chin Up Exercise

This exercise helps eliminate the double chin.

- To begin with, stand upright and maintain your spine straight.

- Then tilt your head towards the back and gaze in the direction of the ceiling.

- Try to imagine you want to kiss the ceiling and then hold this pose for a few seconds.

- Repeat the exercise approximately 15 times daily. In case you have a strain in the neck, avoid the exercise.

Rolling The Neck:

This workout helps remove the double chin by reducing the excess fat accumulated in the chin. It can help tone your chin and jawline too.

- First, stand straight or sit comfortably.

- Then begin to bend your face in one direction. While **aligning your neck** with your chin, start turning your head in a circular motion.

- Ensure you keep your spine straight and the shoulders do not move.

- Repeat the workout in the other direction. You should do the exercise for 5 minutes every day.

Keeping The Tongue Out

This facial workout helps eliminate the double chin.

- Begin by opening your mouth wide and then remove the tongue from the mouth.

- Ensure you're sticking out the tongue as far as possible.

- Then gently bring back the tongue and repeat the workout 10 to 20 times a day.

Jaw Release Exercise

To remove fat from your chin and straighten your cheekbones, try this jaw-releasing workout. The exercise helps stretch the muscles around your jaw, mouth, and lips.

- While sited in a comfortable place, move your mouth as if you want to chew.

- Ensure your lips are fully closed as you exercise.

- Then open your mouth as wide as you can while pressing your tongue to the bottom of your teeth.

- Hold the pose for about 5 seconds and then do five repetitions.

Mouthwash Technique:

This workout helps tone your cheeks and remove the double chin.

- Begin by filling your mouth with air.

- Then, move the air from the left corner of your mouth to the right corner as you do with regular mouthwash.

- Repeat the workout for five rounds a day, each repetition being 5 to 10 minutes.

Chewing Gum

This exercise can help tone the face and make it visibly thinner and younger. All you need is to chew sugar-free gum for approximately 20 minutes a day. The best timing is 30 minutes after lunch or dinner.

Exercises for the Whole Face

The best way to relax your entire face is to try a progressive relaxation exercise that targets all parts of your face, right from the forehead to the chin!

Here's how to get started:

All-over face tone

- Put your hands together in a flat fist, then place your chin over the hands while pressing firmly to create some resistance. This resistance helps maintain your elbows and arms tucked. Hold the pose for a good count of 5 seconds.

- Then squeeze most of the muscles in your face, tuck your chin to your chest, pucker your lips and squint your eyes as you increase the resistance under your chin.

- Alternate this pose with the opposite exercise where you expand rather than contract your face muscles.

- At this point, slowly start lifting your eyes, opening your mouth wide, arching your elbows up, and slightly lifting your chin.

- Hold this position for a count of 3 to 5 seconds.

Fish Face

This workout helps shape your lips, cheeks, and jaws.

- First, close your lips quite softly.

- Then draw your cheeks inwards as much as you can to create a fish face.

- Try to smile as you hold the pose for approximately 15 seconds.

- Relax and try repeating this exercise for five rounds.

Puppet Face

This workout is for the entire face. It helps make your cheek muscles stronger, ensuring they don't become loose.

- Position the tip of your fingers at the point where your cheeks crinkle on your face while smiling.

- Then push your checks up, and now hold the smile.

- Maintain this pose for about 30 seconds, then return to the initial pose.

Face Stretches

This exercise helps relax your face muscles and reduce possible sourness, especially after a full day of facial exercises.

- Whether seated or standing, relax your shoulders and now open your eyes and mouth as much as you can. This helps to stretch the cheeks.

- Maintain this pose for around 20 seconds and return to the initial pose.

The Lion Face

This effective face exercise also helps relax the entire face. This tension reliever helps stretch the entire face and greatly boosts facial blood circulation. The key to this exercise is to ensure that you are sitting straight and taking deep breaths, which makes the exercise more effective.

- First, sit upright and take a deep relaxing breath.

- Then try constricting everything. As you inhale, try tensing most of the muscle groups in the body.

- To make the line face, gently relax your muscles as you breathe out, stick the tongue out and open the eyes as wide as possible. Then splay your hands quite wide.

- Ensure the tongue doesn't just stay out straight; rather, point it downwards as you open your mouth wide or **as if** you're grinning.

- Hold this pose for about 5 to 10 seconds. While doing the exercise, ensure your eyes are wide open to get the maximum benefit from the exercise.

- Relax your entire body and repeat the workout for at least three additional reps. On the last round, try holding the pose for up to 60 seconds.

Face Massage

This is one of the simplest ways to reduce cheek fat, tone, and sculpt your face. Be aware that the excess fluid build-up in the face region brings about the swelling of your neck and face. The good news is that doing regular face massage using therapeutic grade oils such as ginseng oil or wheat germ oil can be a very effective remedy.

These oils help stimulate optimal blood circulation and decrease water retention by draining lymphatic build-up throughout your face.

To do the face massage technique, you can follow these steps:

- Begin by applying wheat germ oil on both your face and neck area.

- Then, gently move your palms in a regular upward direction.

- Start massaging your chin and then slowly move upwards in a gentle circular motion. Repeat this move five more times.

- Next, while using your fingertips, slowly tap from the corners of your lips and carefully move to the direction of your ear.

- Repeat the last step ten times or so.

- At this point, gently move all your fingers except the thumb together with your jawline while using firm and upward stroking movement.

- Repeat this about 5 to 6 times.

Blowing Air Exercise

The exercise helps work out most of the facial and neck muscles. For instance, it can help reduce a double chin and those chubby cheeks since it exercises the cheeks, jaws, and neck muscles.

The workout also helps tone the facial muscles to give you a natural facelift, giving you a leaner facial appearance.

- Begin while sited on a chair with your spine straight.

- Then tilt your head back as far as possible until you're now facing the ceiling, and then pull your lips and slowly exhale.

- Hold this pose for 10 seconds, then relax.

- Repeat for another ten times or so.

After Care

As soon as you're done with the entire face workout, allow your face to obtain enough oxygen by stretching your mouth to the maximum. After a few seconds, relax.

- Take a deep breath and then hold it for a couple of seconds.

- You can then apply a light moisturizer to your hands and rub it on your face.

- Pinch your chicks to obtain a natural red rosy look, and boost blood flow.

How Long Does It Take to See Results?

Adopting this all-natural facial workout regimen can help plump up volume loss in many people. Usually, you're likely to experience a few changes after 3 to 4 days, but you may need up to 3 weeks to notice a more pronounced outcome. In some cases, you might notice "instant results" if doing a series of these exercises a few minutes, say before going on the runway. This will vary from one person to another.

For people concerned that facial exercises might cause more wrinkles, the truth is you hardly workout for as long as you get wrinkles from, say, drinking from a straw.

The rule of the thumb is to relax your eyes and other parts of the face, then focus on your cheek muscles. Within a few days of practice, you should notice which muscle you should be working on.

3 Weeks Facial Exercises Challenge

To help get started on choosing various exercises for whichever day, here is a three-week facial exercises challenge:

Week 1

Day 1

- **Exercise 1:** All-over face tone

Hold the pose for a count of 3 to 5 seconds.

- **Exercise 2:** Double chin workout

Repeat for a set of 5 rounds, each 25 to 30 seconds of tongue holding.

- **Exercise 3:** Jawline workout

Repeat this workout about ten times

Day 2

- **Exercise 1:** Cheekbone lift

Repeat for about 10 to 15 times

- **Exercise 2:** Fish Lips

Do four repetitions in a day

- **Exercise 3:** Eye-firming cheek plumper

Hold for a count of 5 and do 3 to 5 repetitions.

Day 3

- **Exercise 1:** Forehead fine-tuning

Do 8 to 10 times a day for a few weeks

- **Exercise 2:** Wink n' Hold

Repeat for 20 to 25 times per set

- **Exercise 3:** Kiss Face

Repeat for a total of 4 times a day

Day 4

- **Exercise 1:** Cheek plumping

Repeat for 2 to 3 minutes with well-spaced rests.

- **Exercise 2:** Jaw-line defined

Repeat for about 5 reps

- **Exercise 3:** Fish Face

Repeat for 5 rounds

Day 5

- **Exercise 1:** The X and O exercise

Repeat for 10 times

- **Exercise 2:** Cheek squeeze

Repeat for 10 to 15 sets of 5 seconds per round

- **Exercise 3:** The Whistler

Repeat for about 4 times a day

Day 6

- **Exercise 1:** Brow raiser

Repeat for 6 sets of 10 brows raises and drops

- **Exercise 2:** "Rubber" Exercise for forehead

Repeat for about 20 rounds

- **Exercise 3:** Eye toning

Repeat for 6 additional times

Day 7

- **Exercise 1:** Lips workout

Repeat for about 10 times

- **Exercise 2:** The cheek lift

Hold for about 10 seconds

- **Exercise 3:** Neck workout and Neck Stretches

Repeat the neck exercises 3 times.

Week 2

Day 8

- **Exercise 1:** "Hooligan" for Double Chin

Repeat for 5 rounds in each direction

- **Exercise 2:** Puppet face

Hold the pose for 30 seconds

- **Exercise 3:** Saxophone cheeks

Repeat for a total of 10 times

Day 9

- **Exercise 1:** Mandibular exercise for double chin

Hold the pose for 5 seconds.

- **Exercise 2:** Lines around Your Nose

Repeat on the other side

- **Exercise 3:** Droopy eyes and crow's feet exercise

Repeat for a set of 5 rounds

Day 10

- **Exercise 1:** Forehead Push with your hands

Repeat the exercise for 10 rounds

- **Exercise 2:** Neck Mobilization workout

Repeat for 10 times in each direction

- **Exercise 3:** Eyes workout

Repeat once

Day 11

- **Exercise 1:** Squeeze your lips

Repeat for another 3 times

- **Exercise 2:** Puffy Cheeks Exercise

Repeat for 10 times

- **Exercise 3:** Jawline pose

Do 5 to 10 repetitions

Day 12

- **Exercise 1:** Chin Lifts

Repeat for a total of 10 times.

- **Exercise 2:** Face stretches

Hold the pose for 20 seconds

- **Exercise 3:** Chin up exercise

Repeat for 15 times daily.

Day 13

- **Exercise 1:** Rolling the neck

Repeat once for 5 minutes every day

- **Exercise 2:** Blow Balloons

Repeat for another 10 times

- **Exercise 3:** Midface pose

Do 6 to 8 repetitions

Day 14

- **Exercise 1:** Neck and Shoulders Stretches

Hold for a count of 10, then start again

- **Exercise 2:** Frown Line Smoother

Repeat once

- **Exercise 3:** The Forehead Palm Stroke

Repeat the exercise as many times

Week 3

Day 15

- **Exercise 1:** The Flirty Eyes For Brows

Hold for 30 seconds

- **Exercise 2:** Fuller Lips Workout

Repeat for 5 more rounds

- **Exercise 3:** Stretch Your Face Muscles

Repeat 3 times a day

Day 16

- **Exercise 1:** Forehead and Eyes Exercise

Repeat for about 10 rounds

- **Exercise 2:** Shoulder Rolls

Repeat for 10-15 times, and then switch directions

- **Exercise 3:** Keeping the tongue out

Repeat for 10 to 20 times a day

Day 17

- **Exercise 1:** The Lion Face

Repeat for at least 3 additional reps

- **Exercise 2:** Jaw release exercise

Do 5 repetitions

- **Exercise 3:** Rotating Tongue Exercise

Do 15 times in both directions

Day 18

- **Exercise 1:** Upper lip exercise

Do around 5 to 10 reps

- **Exercise 2:** Eyebrows Focus

Repeat for another 4 rounds

- **Exercise 3:** The Forehead Walk

Repeat for a round of 30 seconds

Day 19

- **Exercise 1:** Eyebrow Stretch

Repeat for 5 rounds, and then shut your eyes for 15 seconds.

- **Exercise 2:** Lip Pull

Repeat the exercise once

- **Exercise 3:** Hot Towel Treatment

Repeat for 5 times, 1 hour before bedtime

Day 20

- **Exercise 1:** Forehead pose

Do 5 to 10 repetitions

- **Exercise 2: Face Massage**

Repeat the last step 10 times

- **Exercise 3:** Chewing Gum

Do for 20 minutes a day, 30 minutes after meals.

Day 21

- **Exercise 1:** Mouthwash technique

Repeat for 5 rounds of 5 to 10 minutes each a day

- **Exercise 2:** Blowing Air Exercise

Repeat for 10 times

- **Exercise 3:** Smooth The Brow For Forehead

Repeat for 10 rounds

Face Yoga for Firmer, Toned Skin

Like ordinary yoga, practicing face yoga exercises can make your facial skin look better. According to a 2018 research[3] study, practicing face yoga for 30 minutes a day for eight weeks helps you look three years younger.

We have 43 muscles in our faces, and working them out helps boost blood flow and reduces tension but can strengthen any loose skin. Face yoga comes in handy since it's often harder to target face and neck with normal workouts or even medical treatments.

Unlike various facial exercises, face yoga aims to relax and tone the face. In so doing, it helps combat the negative effects of strained facial expressions to leave your face both rejuvenated and relaxed.

Facial yoga employs exercises and massage techniques that ultimately make loose skin tighter. Studies[4] show that doing facial yoga can help boost the volume around the cheeks,

---

[3] https://jamanetwork.com/journals/jamadermatology/article-abstract/2666801?redirect=true

[4] https://www.mdpi.com/2079-9284/7/1/10

upper lips, and jawline while reducing the appearance of wrinkles and saggy skin.

Facial Yoga Benefits

In addition to toning or slimming the face to counteract aging, other benefits of facial yoga include:

1. *Improves confidence*

Aging signs like facial lines and wrinkles negatively impact personal confidence. By practicing facial yoga, it's possible to tighten facial skin and reduce signs of aging, which goes a long way in restoring confidence.

2. *Boosts overall well being*

Yoga can be extremely soothing and therapeutic! In addition to improving self-esteem, facial yoga helps lower stress levels and boosts your overall physical and mental well-being. This is particularly important in women as looking good also makes them feel better.

3. *It's a natural facelift*

You may have heard about facelift, an expensive face tightening procedure that ultimately helps tighten the skin and make you look younger. However, you don't need to undergo a cosmetic procedure to look younger. Face yoga helps tighten facial muscles and minimize facial lines and wrinkles to create a natural tighter and firmer skin.

4. *You save a lot*

Most cosmetic procedures that provide face tightening options are invasive and financially demanding. Through face yoga, you can save lots of time and money while achieving a healthier, active lifestyle that keeps lifestyle diseases at bay.

The rule of the thumb with facial yoga is to stretch a few minutes in the morning or evening and learn how to control your breath. Here are a few tips to observe before getting started with facial yoga:

How To Prepare For Face Yoga

First, be properly hydrated and relaxed, particularly for the face, neck, and shoulders. Initial warm-up exercises are also important as they put your mind and mind into a safe transition for the facial yoga practice.

As a beginner, you might require warm-up poses for your entire exercising session. Thus, do not shy away from doing them this entire week. The exercises should open your shoulder muscles, groin, lower back, neck, and spine.

Here's a whole-body yoga warm-up sequence you can either do alone or combine with other warm-up exercises.

Ensure you use gentle fluid moments well synced with slow deep breathing. To realize deeper and more effective results, you can hold each stretch for about 1-2 breaths. However, take care if you suffer injuries in the neck, arms, and back because it can worsen the problem.

Here are the most recommended steps to undertake before experimenting with face yoga:

1. *Moisturize and warm up your skin*

It's recommendable to apply a good layer of moisturizer before doing face yoga to keep your face supple while stretching. You can try using a lightweight serum, followed by a pat on eye cream, and finish off with a thin layer of face cream.

- To warm up, tap your fingertips with medium pressure from your forehead to your neck while ensuring you cover all parts of your face.

- Then stretch your head and neck backward and forward.

- Once done, open your mouth as wide as possible to stretch it, and then close the mouth around three times. Doing so helps a lot in relaxing your entire facial muscles.

2. *Try a few deep breathing exercises*

Being calm and relaxed is necessary for most facial exercises. But if you cannot calm down as instantly, you can try a few breathing exercises such as breathing deeply for a count of 4 to 5 seconds. Deep breathing can be a favorite way to meditate before getting into face yoga.

To get started in deep breathing, you can follow these steps:

- Sit on the floor or your bed with your legs crossed.

- Put the right hand down on the bed behind you and then place the left hand on the right knee.

- Sit up straight and deeply breathe in for 4-8 counts, trying to lengthen your spine as you breathe.

- Then begin exhaling as you twist toward the right hand, ensuring that you don't strain the neck.

- Hold this pose for five full breaths, and lengthen the spine on the inhale.

- Ensure you deepen the twist on the exhales if you're comfortable with it. If necessary, you can repeat on the other side.

Belly breathing exercise

- Place one hand on your belt-line, and the other over the chest, just on top of your breastbone. You should easily feel the part of your body or the muscles used in breathing.

- Open the mouth and then let out a gentle sigh, allowing your shoulders and your body muscles to relax as you exhale. The sigh relaxes your upper body muscles but does not fully empty your lungs.

- Now keep your mouth closed and then pause for about 15 seconds. With the mouth closed, inhale slowly through the nose, ensuring that you push your stomach outwards as you breathe. Your belly movement should slightly precede your inhalation as this breathing motion pulls in the air.

- Inhale as much air as possible, and ensure not to throw your upper body into it. When done, now stop with the inhalation exercise.

- Pause for as long as you can, depending on your comfort or lung size. Remember that as you breathe through this technique, you inhale larger portions of air. Therefore, you should breathe more gradually as you normally do. Taking shallow and small breaths can result in lightheadedness that may result in yawning. If you feel lightheaded, slow down as this is just normal.

- Open your mouth, and then slowly exhale through your mouth. As you breathe out, pull your belly in. Now pause and continue practicing steps 3-6.

The measured breath

Here's how you do it:

- Soften up a little, and then choose to either sit or stand. Ensure you relax your hands and also soften your knees. Now drop your shoulders and then allow your jaw to relax.

- At this position, breathe in slowly through the nose. Start to count from 1-4, and keep your shoulders down. Ensure your stomach can expand as you breathe in. Try to hold your breath for a few seconds.

- When done, slowly release your breath very smoothly, as you do a count of 1-7. Repeat this technique for about 10-15 minutes.

Touch the Sky

This beginner deep breathing workout prepares you for more intense exercises and helps you coordinate and control your breathing with each movement.

- Begin seated up straight, preferably in a chair. Position your hands in your lap, and position your palms upwards, while the fingertips point each other.

- Then slowly but deeply breathe in, while raising your hands towards your chest level.

- Shift your palms outward, and now raise your hands over your head. Make sure you aren't reaching too far with your arms; you only need to keep the elbows quite relaxed and bent.

- Relax your arms further as you slowly and deeply breathe out. You should gradually lower the arms to your sides.

- Once down with the breathing exercise, return your hands to the initial pose: the palms facing upward.

- Now repeat the touch the sky exercise about 10 times or so.

3. *Do Muscular Relaxation Exercises*

These are face, neck, and shoulder exercises that can help boost relaxation. You can practice muscular relaxation everywhere, whether in your home, at a desk in your job, or on the road. In the process, ensure you don't get sleepy by toning down each relaxation step to a few seconds that you can maintain.

- Now lie on your back or sit in a well-supported seat if you cannot lie down. Be comfortable, either by lying on a firm bed, probably with some cushions, and then keep your eyes shut.

- Now start working on each of your various muscles groups. Tense each muscle as much as possible, and then relax them completely. Ensure you breathe in when you tense the muscles and out as you relax the muscles.

- Start by concentrating on your breathing for about 5 minutes, and then breathe slowly and smoothly. As

97

you breathe each time, you can try repeating words or phrases such as 'peace' or 'relax.' When done, start relaxing each of your muscles, ensuring that you work on most of the muscle groups around your face, neck, and shoulder areas.

Here is an illustrated stretches guide on how to relax these areas:

Neck

- Get into a comfortable posture, and then start pressing your head back as hard as you can bear.

- Now slowly roll from side to side, and then relax the neck.

- At this point, take a deep breath, hold it for a few seconds and then relax.

- When done with the procedure, return to your normal breathing.

Shoulders

Shoulders are delicate body parts; stretching them can help relieve pain and boost mobility and flexibility.

To do shoulder stretch, follow the following steps:

- Stand shoulder-width apart, and then raise your right arm to the shoulder height.

- Move the arm across the front of your body. Pull the right arm very close to the chest with your left arm.

- Hold for a moment, then switch arms and repeat.

- To complete the shoulder stretch, do 3 to 5 sets of 30 seconds each.

- Once done, finish the relaxation exercise with "Shoulder Clocks."

- Just roll to either side and stack your upper shoulder directly on the lower shoulder.

- Start to make large circles using your upper arm in a clockwise movement. Ensure that the elbow is fully straight as your arm moves in a circular motion.

- Complete 10 repetitions and then switch to the opposite direction. Now repeat on the opposite arm.

After achieving relaxation in the face, neck, and shoulders, it's time to try out the face yoga poses. Here are some of the most recommended exercises.

Face Yoga Poses

Forehead Wrinkles Remover Pose

This pose relaxes the frontalis muscle and reduces tension in your forehead.

- Begin by making a fist with both hands and then position your hands in the center of your forehead.

- Apply some pressure on the forehead, and then slide your fists to the sides.

- Repeat the pose another 4 times.

"Eleven" Lines Yoga Pose

This asana relaxes your corrugator supercilii and procerus muscle, which helps lower tension that brings the 11 lines in between your eyebrows.

- Then put the middle and index finger at the innermost corner of your eyebrows.

- Apply quite some firm pressure, and then spread your fingers slightly apart in a horizontal direction.

- Now take a deep breath and gradually frown as you slowly exhale to a count of 5 seconds.

- Try experiencing the resistance of the muscles located under your fingertips. The idea here is not to try too hard but instead ensure your forehead is fully relaxed.

Crow's-Feet Yoga Pose

This pose helps workout the lower section and the outer corners of your orbicularis oculi muscle and can help reduce the fine lines that form around your eyes.

- First, place the index and middle finger just above your temples, adjacent to your hairline, and then pull upwards. Pause and experience the stretching feeling.

- Now squint without moving your forehead for approximately 5 seconds, then relax.

- Repeat the pose for another 3 rounds.

Laugh Lines Pose (Nasolabial Folds)

This asana helps workout your zygomaticus minor and major muscle, smoothing your nasolabial fold lines.

- Put your palms on your temples and pull up.

- Form an O shape on the mouth while stretching your face long simultaneously

- Then press your upper mouth quite firmly against your teeth.

- Hold the asana for approximately 5 seconds and then relax

- Repeat this move another 3 times.

- Ensure your shoulders are fully relaxed, and now take a few deep inhalations.

The OO-EE Mouth Yoga Pose

This exercise targets the muscles between your nose and the upper lip. The concept here is to make extreme facial movements while making a few sounds.

- First, open your mouth, then pulse both lips together in a way that the teeth are separated but invisible.

- Now say an "OO" sound with an extreme movement to purse the lips together.

- Then, change the sounds to the letters "EE," through an exaggerated motion to fully stretch your lips to the required shape.

- At this point, replace the "EE" sound with the "AH" sound to achieve various ranges of exercises.

- Aim to do approximately 10 repetitions per each different sound for a set of 3 rounds.

The V Exercise

This exercise helps reduce the appearance of forehead wrinkles, along with drooping eyelids, baggy eyes, and crow's feet. Try doing the exercise alongside other facial exercises for your anti-aging ritual.

- To do the exercise, assume you want to make a "V shape" or "peace sign" with both the index and middle fingers in both hands.

104

- Now, use the V shape to frame each of your eyes. Just move the fingers to the point that each eye is in the middle of each V sign. Here, your middle fingers should be under the bridge of your nose, just close to the corner of each eye.

- Meanwhile, set your index fingers such that they touch the outer corner of each upper eyelid. This pose should appear as if you're trying to hold the eyes open with your index and middle finger.

- Check yourself on the mirror if your fingers are forming a V sign below each of your eyes.

- Then gaze up the ceiling as you do a hard squinting with both eyes.

- Using the V shape from the fingers, push the eyes upwards as you squint. Doing so helps workout your forehead muscles and eyebrows against the resistance of the fingers.

- At this point, squeeze your eyes shut. Just move your fingers and try squeezing the eyes shut tightly. Hold the pose for around 10 seconds and then release the pose.

- Relax for a few seconds and repeat the exercise for another 6 rounds while ensuring you squeeze your eyes shut and get enough relaxation in between reps.

Employing the Owl

First, make a C shape using each hand. To do so, visualize yourself holding a pair of binoculars close to your eyes.

- Ensure your thumbs are below your eyes and the index fingers are set just over your brows.

- Now, pull the skin on your forehead using your index fingers to apply strong pressure against the forehead.

- Try raising your brows and opening both your eyes wide. It will require that you work against your fingers for this to be possible.

- Hold this pose for about 2 to 5 seconds to apply downward pressure on the eyes.

- Move the hands from the eyebrows and relax for a few seconds. Then repeat the exercise another three times or so.

- Hold the pose for approximately 10 seconds because it can help tighten and straighten your forehead muscles.

- Do the exercise daily alongside other facial yoga workouts for a line-free forehead to achieve optimum results.

Smoothing the Brow

This exercise can work similarly to Botox because it greatly helps reduce horizontal forehead wrinkles. It also serves as a recommendable recovery workout after a series of other exercises.

- To do this pose, you'll need to rest your hands lightly on your forehead. Ensure that your fingers point inward and face each other.

- Then swipe the fingers outward along your forehead. Apply firm pressure on the skin as you move the fingers from the middle of the forehead to the temples. This helps smooth out the forehead.

- Do not be shy of applying strong pressure on the forehead; you need to feel a firm resistance from the skin.

- Briefly relax your facial muscles and then do a total of 10 reps daily. You may need to pair the exercise with other exercises to see quick results.

Jalandhar Bandha (Chin Lock)

This yoga pose helps shape your face and tones your jawline and facial muscles. It's useful if you have a double chin too.

- First, sit down in the lotus pose, and inhale deeply.

- Then position your hands on your knees, and lift the shoulders as you bend forward.

- At this point, strongly press your chin against the space between the collar bones and the chest then close the food pipe.

- Then try holding your breath as much as you can.

- Now release, take a rest and then repeat the workout.

Neck and Jawline Yoga Pose

This pose helps work out your sternocleidomastoid and platysma muscles to facilitate tightening up your jawline and neck.

- First, turn your chin at a 45-degree angle to the upper right side

- Then pucker the mouth as if you want to kiss. Hold this movement for about 5 seconds, and then relax.

- Repeat the workout on the left side.

Cooldown

Follow these steps below to finish the face yoga workout with all your facial muscles relaxed fully.

- Tap your fingertips with both hands from the top of your forehead down to your neck.

- Repeat this another 3 times or so.

Tips On How To Do Face Yoga Exercises

- It's advisable to do the yoga exercises in front of the mirror to assess whether you're doing things right or not.

- Calm down. As a beginner, you'll need to remain calm and relaxed to facilitate slow and steady progress.

- When exercising, ensure your face, neck, and shoulders are fully relaxed.

- Take care of your eyes, don't press them so hard or forcefully massage the skin such that it can fold itself.

- Make sure you wash your hands before facial exercises, as touching the face may add dirt and oils that further bring breakouts.

- Choose a **fixed number of exercises** to do before you go to sleep every night, and shuffle the rest of the exercises in various workouts.

To help get started on choosing various exercises for whichever day, here is a 28 days facial yoga workout challenge:

28 Day Facial Yoga Program

Week 1

Day 1

- **Exercise:** Forehead Wrinkles Remover Pose

Repeat for 4 times

Day 2

- **Exercise:** "Eleven" Lines Yoga Pose

Repeat once

Day 3

- **Exercise:** Crow's-Feet Yoga Pose

Repeat for another 3 rounds

Day 4

- **Exercise:** Laugh Lines Pose

Repeat for another 3 times

Day 5

- **Exercise:** The OO-EE Mouth Yoga Pose

Do 10 repetitions per round, for a set of 3 rounds

Day 6

- **Exercise:** The V exercise

Repeat the exercise for another 6 rounds

Day 7

- **Exercise:** Employing the Owl

Repeat another 3 times

Week 2

Day 8

- **Exercise:** Smoothing the Brow

Do a total of 10 reps daily

Day 9

- **Exercise:** Jalandhar Bandha (Chin Lock)

Repeat the pose once

Day 10

- **Exercise:** Neck and Jawline Yoga pose

Repeat on the other side

Day 11

- **Exercise:** Forehead Wrinkles Remover Pose

Repeat for 4 times

Day 12

- **Exercise:** "Eleven" Lines Yoga Pose

Repeat once

Day 13

- **Exercise:** Crow's-Feet Yoga Pose

Repeat for another 3 rounds

Day 14

- **Exercise:** Laugh Lines Pose

Repeat for another 3 times

Week 3

Day 15

- **Exercise:** The OO-EE Mouth Yoga Pose

Do 10 repetitions per round, for a set of 3 rounds

Day 16

- **Exercise:** The V exercise

Repeat the exercise for another 6 rounds

Day 17

- **Exercise:** Employing the Owl

Repeat for another 3 times

Day 18

- **Exercise:** Smoothing the Brow

Do a total of 10 reps daily

Day 19

- **Exercise:** Jalandhar Bandha (Chin Lock)

Repeat the pose once

Day 20

- **Exercise:** Neck and Jawline Yoga pose

Repeat on the other side

Day 21

- **Exercise:** Forehead Wrinkles Remover Pose

Repeat for 4 times

Week 4

Day 22

- **Exercise:** "Eleven" Lines Yoga Pose

Repeat once

Day 23

- **Exercise:** Crow's-Feet Yoga Pose

Repeat for another 3 rounds

Day 24

- **Exercise:** Laugh Lines Pose

Repeat for another 3 times

Day 25

- **Exercise:** The OO-EE Mouth Yoga Pose

Do 10 repetitions per round, for a set of 3 rounds

Day 26

- **Exercise:** The V exercise

Repeat the exercise for another 6 rounds

Day 27

- **Exercise:** Employing the Owl

Repeat for another 3 times

Day 28

- **Exercise:** Smoothing the Brow

Do a total of 10 reps daily

Taking Care of Your Face

Here're a few tips that will help you take care of your now-youthful looking face:

Smile as much as you can

Like facial exercises, smiling can strengthen your face muscles and make you appear admirable when exercising. Smiling also helps boost confidence and relaxation, particularly when working in a stressful environment.

Keep your face clean

It's advisable to wash the face regularly and keep the skin clear of impurities. You can add a moisturizer, face cleanser, or retinoid to your washing if need be. However, make the routine activity very simple as too many skincare products may produce unexpected results.

Eat well for strong skin

Even though facial exercises can tighten the skin and make you look younger, your face needs a nutrition boost. Nutrients such as vitamins A and C and organic sources of omega 3 fatty acids can help maintain your face muscles well developed and your skin clear.

You can try other foods like dark-colored veggies and leafy fruits like spinach, carrots, beans, tomatoes, and blueberries. Add in omega 3 rich foods such as salmon, mackerel, and raw dark chocolate.

The rule of the thumb is to get organic or unprocessed healthy foods while avoiding those high refined carbohydrates and high-fat foods that encourage premature skin aging.

Protect your face from the sun

Exposure to direct sunlight will further damage your face or give you a more aging look. If working outdoors during peak sunlight hours of 10 am to 2 pm, get clothing that can cover your body well and apply sunscreen.

Try essential oils massage

Applying essential oils on the skin triggers the release of biochemical sensors that send signals that lower cell inflammation. Based on various studies[5], the body massage technique helps cells make new mitochondrial cells, which helps boost power-production centers within face cells.

You can use a wide variety of essential oils such as lemon oil and lavender directly on the face skin areas such as the forehead, cheeks, neck, and chin. For instance, you can massage 1-3 drops of oil on the desired area in a circular motion to increase the oil's effectiveness.

When doing a full face massage, mix around 6 drops of oil with a different lotion and then do any suitable hand massage technique. Then do a repeated rubbing so that the skin can fully absorb the oil.

You can use a localized massage[6] when targeting small areas that are uncomfortable or aching, such as stiff jaws and facial muscle sprains. Ensure you dilute about 10 drops of oil with one teaspoon of carrier oil.

---

[5] https://www.sciencebasedmedicine.org/massage-therapy-decreases-inflammation/

[6] https://www.visitlescala.com/en/to-do/health-beauty/localized-massage

If doing a facial massage for the first time, take care not to have the oil get into contact with your eyes, nose, or mouth and use a lower dose than that of other facial area massages. For instance, you can use 1-3 drops of oil with a teaspoon of carrier oil, or even less if you're sensitive to oils.

Conclusion

As you have seen, there are many ways of working out your facial muscles for that toned, youthful look. It's now your time to try most of these easy exercises from Mother Nature's gift of face yoga and facial exercises.

Good luck!

PS: I'd like your feedback. If you are happy with this book, please leave a review on Amazon.

Please leave a review for this book on Amazon by visiting the page below:

https://amzn.to/2VMR5qr